COMPLETE GUIDE TO
EPILEPSY SURGERY

Comprehensive Handbook To Advanced Techniques, Patient Care, And Post-Surgical Outcomes

DR. BRUNO HORAN

Copyright © 2023 by Dr. Bruno Horan

All rights reserved. Except for brief quotations embodied in critical reviews and certain other noncommercial uses permitted by copyright law, no part of this publication may be reproduced, distributed, or transmitted in any form or by any means, Including photocopying, recording, or other electronic or mechanical methods, without the prior written permission of the publisher.

Disclaimer:

The information provided in this book, is intended for general informational purposes only and should not be considered as professional advice.

The author has made every effort to ensure the accuracy of the information presented. However, readers are advised to consult with a qualified healthcare professional before attempting any herbal remedies or making significant changes to their wellness routine. Individual health conditions vary, and what may be suitable for one person may not be appropriate for another.

It is important to note that the author is not in any endorsement deal, partnership, or affiliation with any organization, brand, or company mentioned in this book. Any references to specific products or services are based on the author's personal experience or general knowledge and do not imply an endorsement or promotion of those products or services

Contents

CHAPTER ONE 13
  SYNOPSIS OF EPILEPSY 13
    The Meaning And Categorization Of Epilepsy 13
    Reasons And Danger Elements 14
    Signs And Types Of Seizures 15
    Procedures For Diagnosis 16
    Effect On Life Quality 17

CHAPTER TWO 19
  EPILEPSY: MEDICAL MANAGEMENT 19
    Aeds, Or Anti-Epileptic Medications 19
    Non-Pharmacological Interventions 20
    Dietary And Lifestyle Adjustments 21
    Keeping An Eye On And Controlling Adverse Consequences 22
    Assessing The Efficacy Of Treatment 22

CHAPTER THREE 25
  MEDICATION INDICATIONS 25
    Standards For Examining Surgery 26
    Assessment Of Medical Unpredictability 27

Genetics's Contribution To Surgical Decision-Making 28

Social And Psychological Evaluations.................29

Extended Outlook Absent Surgery 30

CHAPTER FOUR 31

BEFORE SURGERY, EVALUATIONS 31

A Thorough Physical Examination And Medical History 31

Superior Imaging Methods 32

Monitoring: Invasive And Non-Invasive 32

Maps Of The Brain In Function 33

Assessment Of Multidisciplinary Teams 34

CHAPTER FIVE 35

EPILEPSY SURGERY TYPES...................................35

Reconstructive Surgery 35

Surgery For Disconnection 36

Methods Of Neurostimulation 37

LITT Stands For Laser Interstitial Thermal Therapy..39

New Advances In Surgery 40

CHAPTER SIX..43

THE SURGICAL METHOD 43
   Before Surgery 44
   Roles Of The Anesthesia And Surgical Teams 44
   Methodical Surgical Procedure 45
   Monitoring During Operation 46
   Recovery And Postoperative Care 46
CHAPTER SEVEN 49
  POST-OPTICAL REHABILITATION 49
   Quick Postoperative Treatment 51
   Physical Therapy And Rehabilitation 52
CHAPTER EIGHT 55
  RESULTS AND PREDICTION 55
   Success Rates As Well As Possible Advantages ... 56
   Hazards And Possible Issues 58
   Enhancements In Life Quality 59
   Case Studies And Testimonials From Patients 60
CHAPTER NINE 63
  COMMON QUESTIONS AND ANSWERS 63
   Taking Care Of Often Held Myths And Fears 64
   Faqs Regarding Surgery For Epilepsy 66

Coping Techniques For Families And Patients 67

Financial And Legal Aspects To Take Into Account 68

Sources Of Additional Data And Assistance.........70

ABOUT THE BOOK

"Epilepsy Surgery" is a seminal work in the area that provides a thorough examination of the complexities involved in managing epilepsy with surgery. From its thorough analysis of the definition and categorization of epilepsy to its sophisticated comprehension of its origins, risk factors, and varied symptomatology, the book establishes a solid foundation for both novices and experts. It highlights the need and importance of efficient treatment plans by exploring diagnostic processes and the significant impact of epilepsy on quality of life.

The book's thorough presentation of medical management, which clarifies the function of anti-epileptic medications in addition to non-pharmacological therapies, dietary modifications, and careful monitoring procedures, is its main focus. These kinds of discoveries are priceless because they give medical professionals practical ways to improve patient outcomes and lessen problems associated with therapy.

Its emphasis on surgical indications, which provides precise standards for when surgical intervention is required, is a distinguishing characteristic. It makes precise surgical decisions by navigating the difficulties of pre-operative examinations and utilizing interdisciplinary evaluations and modern imaging tools.

This all-encompassing strategy highlights the book's dedication to fusing medical knowledge with sophisticated patient care.

The book highlights a variety of surgical modalities and explains the nuances of each surgery, ranging from modern neurostimulation techniques and laser interstitial thermal therapy to respective disconnection surgeries. It walks readers through the whole surgical process, stressing thorough patient management at each stage, from painstaking preoperative planning to intraoperative monitoring and aftercare.

Beyond surgical results, post-surgery recovery, rehabilitation techniques, and long-term prognostic factors are covered. Through case studies, patient testimonies, and current research findings, the book highlights how epilepsy surgery can significantly improve quality of life and address unresolved issues.

"Epilepsy Surgery" goes beyond clinical discourse by addressing common worries, legal considerations, and patient support options.

This compassionate dialogue empowers both patients and caregivers. Its integration of patient advocacy, clinical knowledge, and ethical issues highlights its significance as a key tool in influencing the direction of epilepsy treatment going forward, in addition to its role as a textbook.

CHAPTER ONE

SYNOPSIS OF EPILEPSY

Recurrent seizures are the hallmark of epilepsy, a neurological condition brought on by aberrant electrical activity in the brain.

The degree, frequency, and nature of these seizures can vary greatly, making epilepsy a challenging condition to manage. It affects individuals of all ages, from young children to the elderly, and can have a big influence on day-to-day activities and general well-being.

The Meaning And Categorization Of Epilepsy

The definition of epilepsy is a chronic illness characterized by frequent, erratic seizures. The actual seizures are periods of disrupted brain activity brought on by aberrant electrical discharges in the brain. Depending on which area of the brain is affected, these discharges may result in changes in behavior, movements, sensations, or consciousness.

Several aspects are taken into consideration when classifying epilepsy, such as the kind of seizures one has, the underlying cause (if any), and the clinical presentation of the seizures. Two common classifications are focal epilepsy, which originates in one area of the brain, and generalized epilepsy, which affects both hemispheres of the brain. Identification of particular syndromes according to seizure type, age of start, and other clinical characteristics may be necessary for further classification.

Reasons And Danger Elements

There might be a vast range of unknown causes for epilepsy. Genetics, brain tumors, illnesses that damage the brain (meningitis, for example), trauma or stroke, developmental abnormalities (cerebral palsy, for example), and infections are other common reasons. However, in many situations, the cause of idiopathic epilepsy is still unknown.

A family history of the condition, head trauma, brain infections, prenatal trauma or developmental abnormalities, and specific genetic conditions are risk factors for developing epilepsy. Knowing these risk factors can occasionally assist in identifying people who may be more prone to epilepsy development.

Signs And Types Of Seizures

Depending on the kind of seizure, epilepsy symptoms can range from mild to severe. Both sides of the brain are affected by generalized seizures, which can result in convulsions, generalized muscle rigidity, or spasms. They can also induce loss of consciousness. Specific brain regions can give rise to focal seizures, which can result in localized symptoms such as altered consciousness, involuntary movements, or sensory disturbances.

The most common types of seizures are myoclonic seizures, which are quick, brief jerks of the muscles, absence seizures, which are momentary loss of awareness, and focal impaired awareness seizures, which were once known as complex partial seizures. It is essential to identify the precise type of seizure to make an accurate diagnosis and develop a treatment plan.

Procedures For Diagnosis

A comprehensive medical history, a neurological examination, and several diagnostic procedures are usually required to diagnose epilepsy. The electroencephalogram (EEG) is a widely used tool for recording electrical activity in the brain and is useful in identifying aberrant patterns that may indicate epilepsy. To find anatomical irregularities or brain lesions that may be the source of seizures, imaging tests like magnetic resonance imaging (MRI) may also be carried out.

To further explore the underlying reason or evaluate cognitive function, other procedures including blood tests, lumbar punctures (spinal taps), or neuropsychological assessments may occasionally be carried out. These diagnostic processes are intended to determine whether epilepsy is present, categorize the kind of seizures, and collect data necessary for creating a successful treatment strategy.

Effect On Life Quality

A person's quality of life can be greatly impacted by having epilepsy. Seizures can be unpredictable, which can make it difficult to carry out everyday tasks like driving, finding work, and interacting with people. Emotional and psychological difficulties may also be exacerbated by a fear of suffering harm during a seizure or of having one in public.

A multidisciplinary strategy combining neurologists, epileptologists, nurses, and other healthcare providers is frequently necessary for managing epilepsy. Antiepileptic drugs, lifestyle changes (including sticking to a regular sleep schedule and avoiding triggers), and in certain situations, surgical intervention are all possible forms of treatment.

Giving people with epilepsy comprehensive treatment and support requires an understanding of how the condition affects their quality of life.

Healthcare practitioners can improve the overall well-being of patients and their families and improve patient outcomes by addressing both the medical and psychosocial elements of epilepsy.

CHAPTER TWO

EPILEPSY: MEDICAL MANAGEMENT

The mainstay of treatment for epilepsy, a neurological condition marked by recurring seizures, is medication intended to minimize and regulate seizure activity. Anti-epileptic drugs (AEDs) are pharmaceuticals that are expressly intended to prevent or reduce the frequency and intensity of seizures. They constitute the cornerstone of medical care.

Aeds, Or Anti-Epileptic Medications

Anti-epileptic medications function by balancing the brain's electrical activity, which lessens the possibility of aberrant electrical discharges that cause seizures. The kind, frequency, and unique medical history of each patient are taken into consideration while prescribing these drugs. To obtain optimal seizure control, patients must closely follow their specified drug regimen.

AEDs come in a variety of classes, each with its specific mode of action and possible adverse effects. Among the medications that are frequently administered include levetiracetam, valproate, lamotrigine, and carbamazepine. The type of epilepsy, the patient's age, and any underlying medical issues all influence the treatment decision.

Non-Pharmacological Interventions

Non-pharmacological therapies can be very helpful in controlling epilepsy in addition to AEDs. Among these are treatments like vagus nerve stimulation (VNS), which entails implanting a gadget to stimulate the vagus nerve in the neck with electrical impulses to assist avoid seizures. Response-based neurostimulation (RNS) is an additional choice in which an implanted device in the brain recognizes and reacts to abnormal electrical activity, thereby averting seizures before they start.

When medicine or other treatments are ineffective for treating a particular case of epilepsy, surgical techniques may also be considered. The goal of epilepsy surgery is to cut off or eliminate the epileptogenic zone—the region of the brain that causes seizures. For some patients, this surgery might completely stop or drastically minimize seizure activity.

Dietary And Lifestyle Adjustments

In addition to drugs and surgery, dietary and lifestyle changes can help treat epilepsy. For example, research has demonstrated that the ketogenic diet, which is low in carbohydrates and high in fats, can effectively reduce seizures, particularly in children who have epilepsy.

In a similar vein, seizure frequency can be reduced by adhering to a normal sleep pattern, controlling stress levels, and avoiding triggers like alcohol or particular foods.

Keeping An Eye On And Controlling Adverse Consequences

Vigilant monitoring and control of any anti-epileptic medication side effects are essential components of effective epilepsy care. Mood swings, weight gain, tiredness, and dizziness are a few typical side effects. It is crucial to schedule routine follow-up visits with healthcare professionals to evaluate the effectiveness of medications, modify dosages as necessary, and quickly address any new side effects.

Assessing The Efficacy Of Treatment

Monitoring the frequency and intensity of seizures over time is necessary to evaluate how well epilepsy treatments are working. To document information about each seizure, including the date, time, duration, and events leading up to it, patients are frequently advised to keep a seizure diary. This data assists medical professionals in determining whether the current course of treatment is effectively controlling seizures or whether changes are required.

Further diagnostic testing, such as an electroencephalogram (EEG), magnetic resonance imaging (MRI), or positron emission tomography (PET) scan, may be necessary to pinpoint the precise regions of aberrant brain activity in cases where seizures continue to occur despite treatment.

With a focus on achieving optimal results in seizure control and quality of life, our all-encompassing approach guarantees that treatment programs are customized to meet the specific needs of each patient.

CHAPTER THREE
MEDICATION INDICATIONS

When medicine is unable to sufficiently control seizures or when the adverse effects of medication are unacceptable, epilepsy surgery may be considered. Drug-resistant epilepsy, commonly referred to as medically intractable epilepsy, is the primary indicator. The standard definition of this syndrome is the inability to attain prolonged seizure independence after two or more trials of antiepileptic drugs that have been carefully selected and tolerated. In such circumstances, surgery aims to drastically reduce the frequency and severity of seizures or to eliminate them.

When seizures originate from a particular, well-defined brain region that may be safely removed without resulting in major neurological damage, it is another clue that epilepsy surgery is warranted.

This is frequently the case with focal epilepsy, in which a limited region of aberrant brain tissue—such as a tumor or a scar from an earlier injury—is the source of the seizures.

Standards For Examining Surgery

Consideration of epilepsy surgery is based on several important factors. To ensure that surgery is appropriate for the particular form of epilepsy, it is first necessary to appropriately diagnose and classify the seizures.

To confirm the presence of drug-resistant epilepsy, a detailed evaluation of the patient's medical history is conducted, including an assessment of the effectiveness and tolerance of antiepileptic medications.

Finding the underlying structural abnormalities in the brain that may be causing seizures requires the use of neuroimaging investigations, such as magnetic resonance imaging (MRI) scans.

Comprehensive neurological exams also aid in identifying the location and kind of the epileptic focal, such as electroencephalograms (EEGs) and neuropsychological tests.

Assessment Of Medical Unpredictability

When two or more antiepileptic medications have been adequately tried and seizures still occur, this is known as medical intractability in epilepsy. It is an important consideration when deciding whether surgery is necessary.

To prove intractability, a thorough record of seizure frequency, kind, and impact on everyday life is required.

Neurologists and epileptologists can use this information to evaluate the pros and cons of surgery in comparison to ongoing medical treatment, as well as to determine the severity of the problem.

Genetics's Contribution To Surgical Decision-Making

The decision to have epilepsy surgery can be greatly influenced by genetics, especially in situations where a known hereditary predisposition to a certain form of epileptic condition exists.

Genetic testing can reveal particular gene variants or mutations that impact treatment options and surgery planning and contribute to the epilepsy phenotype.

Comprehending the hereditary foundation of epilepsy can also aid in forecasting the probability of surgical triumph and the chance of recurrence after surgery.

Genetic testing may occasionally identify disorders linked to an increased risk of developing drug-resistant epilepsy, which may lead to an early assessment of surgical procedures

Social And Psychological Evaluations

The evaluation process for epilepsy surgery includes social and psychological evaluations. Through these evaluations, the patient's social support networks, cognitive and emotional functioning, and capacity to handle the possible hardships of surgery and recuperation are all intended to be evaluated.

Memory, language, attention, and executive function tests are frequently included in psychological examinations.

These tests are essential for determining the possible cognitive hazards connected to surgery. To make sure that patients have access to sufficient resources and help both before and after surgery, social assessments concentrate on the patient's housing arrangement, work status, and support system.

Extended Outlook Absent Surgery

Without surgery, the long-term prognosis for epilepsy varies based on several factors, such as the kind of epilepsy, frequency of seizures, underlying etiology, and treatment response. The prognosis for those with drug-resistant epilepsy who choose not to have surgery could include continuing medication therapy despite continuous seizures, which could result in gradual cognitive deterioration and a lower quality of life.

The objective of attaining seizure independence or considerable reduction in seizures might be more difficult to achieve without surgical intervention. The management of epilepsy becomes more challenging when antiepileptic medicine is used for an extended period due to the possibility of adverse effects and decreased efficacy.

CHAPTER FOUR

BEFORE SURGERY, EVALUATIONS

A Thorough Physical Examination And Medical History

Patients go through a rigorous evaluation process to make sure they are good candidates for epilepsy surgery before having the treatment done.

The medical team first acquires information regarding the patient's seizure frequency, severity, and kinds through a thorough assessment of their medical history.

Knowing the past makes it easier to spot trends that can direct the surgical strategy. A thorough physical examination is also performed to evaluate general health and find any conditions that might affect surgery or recovery.

Superior Imaging Methods

When evaluating patients with epilepsy before surgery, advanced imaging is essential. The structure and function of the brain can be seen using methods like positron emission tomography (PET) scans and magnetic resonance imaging (MRI).

A structural abnormality that may be causing seizures, such as a tumor, lesion, or scar, can be found via magnetic resonance imaging (MRI).

PET scans can assist in identifying regions of aberrant activity that are associated with the beginning of seizures and can reveal information about brain metabolism.

Monitoring: Invasive And Non-Invasive

It is crucial to track brain activity to identify the precise site of seizure onset. Initially, non-invasive techniques such as electroencephalography (EEG) are employed to continuously record brain electrical activity, thereby detecting possible seizure foci and documenting seizure patterns. When non-invasive techniques are unsatisfactory, intrusive monitoring—which entails putting electrodes directly on the brain or inside brain tissue—can be extremely helpful in providing more accurate information regarding the location of seizures.

Maps Of The Brain In Function

A sophisticated method called functional brain mapping is used to pinpoint the precise regions of the brain that are in charge of vital processes like speech, movement, and sensation.

By removing or disconnecting the seizure focus, neurosurgeons can organize the procedure to minimize damage to important brain areas. Intraoperative mapping is one technique where vital functions are retained by monitoring responses in real time throughout the surgery.

Assessment Of Multidisciplinary Teams

To assess and treat each patient completely, a multidisciplinary team of doctors works together during epilepsy surgery.

Neurologists, neurosurgeons, neuropsychologists, neuroradiologists, and specialty nurses usually make up this team.

Every member contributes their distinct area of knowledge to the table, enabling a comprehensive evaluation of the patient's state. They go over every test result, talk about possible courses of action, and create a customized surgical plan based on the needs and objectives of the individual patient.

CHAPTER FIVE

EPILEPSY SURGERY TYPES

Reconstructive Surgery

One type of epilepsy surgery called resection aims to remove or resect the part of the brain that causes seizures. It is usually taken into consideration when a specific and easily accessible area of the brain is the source of the seizures. The two most popular respective surgery procedures are laminectomy and lobectomy.

A lobectomy is the surgical removal of a particular brain lobe that is the source of seizures. To properly locate the epileptic focus, this surgery is meticulously planned utilizing pre-operative imaging tools such as MRI and PET scans.

The goal of a laminectomy is to remove a particular brain lesion or abnormality that is producing seizures. Tumors, scars from prior injuries, and abnormal blood vessels are examples of lesions. The goal of this procedure is to remove the cause of the aberrant electrical activity in the brain.

For patients whose seizures are well-defined and limited to a particular area of the brain, both lobectomy and laminectomy are thought to be beneficial treatments. Proper identification of the epileptic focus and cautious planning to limit influence on critical brain functions are often critical to the success of these procedures.

Surgery For Disconnection

When drugs or other treatments are ineffective in controlling seizures that affect both hemispheres of the brain, disconnecting the brain via surgery, such as corpus callosotomy, is the next step. To stop seizures from spreading from one hemisphere to the other, the corpus callosum—a band of nerve fibers linking the two hemispheres—is cut either whole or partially.

Patients with severe generalized seizures, such as drop attacks (tonic-clonic seizures) that do not react well to medicine, benefit most from corpus callosotomy. With corpus callosotomy, the frequency and intensity of seizures are intended to be decreased by blocking the routes that allow seizures to travel between the hemispheres.

Based on the kind and frequency of seizures a patient has, their overall neurological function, and their quality of life, this procedure is carefully considered. Corpus callosotomy can greatly enhance seizure control and lower the risk of harm during seizures, even while surgery does not completely prevent seizures.

Methods Of Neurostimulation

Implanted devices are used in neurostimulation treatments to control brain activity and lessen seizures. Patients who are not candidates for disconnection or reconstructive surgery or for whom these procedures have not produced adequate seizure control are usually considered these treatments.

For the treatment of epilepsy, one of the most well-known neurostimulation methods is vagus nerve stimulation (VNS). A gadget that stimulates the vagus nerve, which passes through the neck and into the brain, is implanted. Through the regular delivery of electrical impulses to the brain, VNS seeks to lessen both the frequency and severity of seizures.

A more recent method called responsive neurostimulation (RNS) involves implanting a device just where seizures begin, in the brain. To stop seizure activity before it spreads, RNS continuously analyzes brain activity and applies electrical stimulation. The closed-loop system is intended to adapt to the distinct seizure patterns of every patient.

Another neurostimulation method is called Deep Brain Stimulation (DBS), and it entails implanting electrodes into particular brain regions that are known to be involved in the production of seizures. To control aberrant brain activity and lower the frequency of seizures, electrical impulses are administered. DBS is being investigated further for epilepsy and is being considered for patients who have difficult-to-control seizures of a particular type.

LITT Stands For Laser Interstitial Thermal Therapy.

A minimally invasive surgical method called laser interstitial thermal treatment (LITT) is used to treat epilepsy, especially when the epileptic center is situated deep within the brain or in places that are challenging to reach with conventional surgery.

By carefully heating and destroying aberrant brain tissue that causes seizures, LITT uses laser energy.

A tiny hole in the skull is used to introduce a thin laser probe into the target region, which is located using sophisticated imaging methods. After positioning itself, the laser is turned on to minimize harm to the surrounding healthy brain tissue while heating and ablating the epileptic tissue.

Compared to open surgery, LITT has several benefits, such as shorter hospital stays, faster recovery periods, and a lower chance of problems like infection and injury to healthy brain tissue.

Patients who experience seizures originating from key parts of the brain or who may not be able to handle more intrusive procedures would benefit most from it.

New Advances In Surgery

Apart from the well-known procedures for epilepsy, there are continuous improvements in surgical methods targeted at enhancing the results for epilepsy patients.

With less intrusive alternatives to conventional reconstructive procedures like lobectomies and laminectomies, minimally invasive surgery, or MIS, is still developing. MIS procedures minimize surgical trauma and recovery periods by using specialized instruments and smaller incisions guided by sophisticated imaging.

Modern navigation and imaging technology are essential for increasing the accuracy and security of epilepsy procedures.

With the least amount of harm to healthy brain tissue, surgeons can more precisely identify and target epileptic foci thanks to techniques like intraoperative magnetic resonance imaging and neuronavigation systems.

Another new development in epilepsy surgery is robot-assisted surgery, in which robotic devices help doctors conduct precise and deliberate movements while doing operations.

Improved surgical accuracy and better patient outcomes are the goals of this technology, especially in difficult cases.

In terms of treating epilepsy, these cutting-edge surgical methods offer fresh hope for those who have not responded to traditional medications or who need specialized care that is catered to their unique seizure patterns and brain structure.

CHAPTER SIX
THE SURGICAL METHOD

A specialist operation called epilepsy surgery is used to reduce or completely eradicate seizures in people who are not responding to medication. After a comprehensive examination by a multidisciplinary team of neurologists, neurosurgeons, neuropsychologists, and other specialists, the decision to have surgery is frequently made. The precise kind of epilepsy and the location of the seizure focal in the brain determine the surgical technique that is used.

Respective surgery is a popular type of epilepsy surgery in which the epileptic focus (the part of the brain from which seizures originate) is surgically removed. To correctly pinpoint the seizure focal, this operation is carefully planned using preoperative imaging studies, such as MRI and EEG (electroencephalogram). Disconnective surgery is a different kind of surgery where the goal is to stop the abnormal electrical activity from spreading by interrupting the brain circuits that cause seizures.

Before Surgery

To make sure they are good candidates for epilepsy surgery, patients go through a rigorous preoperative screening before surgery. This includes thorough neurological evaluations, cognitive function tests using neuropsychological testing, and exact mapping of the brain areas related to epilepsy using imaging examinations. To maximize care both during and after surgery, the medical staff also looks over the patient's past medical records and current prescriptions.

Roles Of The Anesthesia And Surgical Teams

A proficient anesthetic team is essential to guarantee the patient's safety and comfort during epilepsy surgery.

Throughout the process, anesthesia is carefully given to create unconsciousness and provide pain relief. The delicate operation is carried out by the neurosurgical team, which is headed by a neurosurgeon with expertise in epilepsy surgery. Neurophysiologists assist them by continuously observing brain activity to inform surgical choices.

Methodical Surgical Procedure

Usually, the neurosurgeon makes an exact incision in the scalp to gain access to the skull before starting the surgical procedure.

The neurosurgeon may employ sophisticated imaging methods, such as intraoperative magnetic resonance imaging (MRI) or neuronavigation, to precisely identify and target the seizure focus, depending on the type of operation that is planned.

After the brain is exposed, the identified epileptic focus is carefully removed or disconnected by the neurosurgeon to cause the least amount of damage to the surrounding healthy brain tissue.

Monitoring During Operation

To guarantee both the safety and effectiveness of epilepsy surgery, intraoperative monitoring is essential.

To track brain activity in real-time, neurophysiologists employ a range of methods including direct cortical stimulation, evoked potentials, and electroencephalograms.

This aids in the identification and preservation of important brain regions in charge of speech, movement, and sensation.

The neurosurgeon bases his or her decisions on any abnormal brain activity found during the procedure to maximize results.

Recovery And Postoperative Care

Following surgery, patients are kept under strict observation in either an epilepsy monitoring unit

(EMU) or an intensive care unit (ICU). The priorities are infection control, pain management, and neurological status monitoring.

Depending on where the surgery is being performed, patients may feel temporary weakness, trouble speaking, or other symptoms. Physical therapy and rehabilitation could be required to maximize recovery and assist with function restoration.

CHAPTER SEVEN

POST-OPTICAL REHABILITATION

Immediately following epilepsy surgery, the patient's recuperation becomes the primary priority. This stage starts in the hospital, where doctors keep a careful eye on patients' neurological conditions and vital signs.

Pain management techniques are used to maintain the patient's comfort, frequently using a custom-made drug combination.

The surgical site is also closely watched for any indications of infection or other problems.

To promote healing, healthcare professionals make sure patients have balanced meals and enough water. Nutrition plays a critical role in the healing process.

To provide adequate nourishment and hydration, a temporary feeding tube may be needed initially, depending on the type of surgery performed and the patient's health.

It is advised for family members and caregivers to get involved in the healing process by learning how to help with everyday tasks and being aware of any possible difficulties. The patient's overall healing and emotional health depend on this support system.

To guarantee a seamless transfer from the hospital to home or a rehabilitation facility, discharge planning starts early.

This could entail making plans for physical therapy, home health care, or any necessary follow-up appointments with doctors.

To encourage healing and avoid complications, detailed instructions are given on wound care, medication administration, and any activity restrictions.

Quick Postoperative Treatment

Patients are intensively followed in an intensive care unit or specialist neurosurgery recovery center following epilepsy surgery. During this time, the main objectives are to keep the patient's condition stable, successfully manage their pain, and avoid complications.

To quickly address any potential problems, there is constant monitoring of the surgical site, neurological condition, and vital signs.

When necessary, intravenous fluids and drugs are given to maintain hydration and control discomfort. To keep patients comfortable and to quickly handle any early indications of complications, such as bleeding or infection, nurses and doctors collaborate.

At first, patients can need help with simple tasks like eating, drinking, and getting around. Early intervention by occupational and physical therapists can help patients regain strength and independence. Early mobilization is advised to avoid issues including blood clots and muscle stiffness, under the supervision of medical personnel.

Family members are frequently given information on what to anticipate during this stage and how to assist in the patient's healing. They might learn how to manage medicine, help with wound care, and spot potential consequences. A coordinated approach to care is ensured by the healthcare team and the patient's support system having clear lines of communication.

Physical Therapy And Rehabilitation

Physical therapy and rehabilitation are essential parts of the healing process after epilepsy surgery.

The type of surgery done and the severity of any neurological abnormalities determine the exact rehabilitation approach that is needed for each patient.

The goals of physical therapists are to increase mobility, strength, and balance. To assist patients in regaining their motor skills and coordination, they could introduce exercises, progressively increasing the difficulty as the patient gets better.

Treatment plans are designed to avoid joint stiffness and muscle atrophy while enhancing general physical health.

Occupational therapists assist patients with regaining the abilities needed for everyday tasks including driving, cooking, and self-care.

To maximize freedom and safety, they could suggest modifying the home or recommending adaptable equipment.

If swallowing or speaking has been impacted by the procedure, speech therapists might be involved. In addition to making sure patients can eat and drink safely, they assess patients and offer therapies to enhance communication.

In the weeks and months after surgery, rehabilitation sessions are usually planned regularly to track recovery and make any modifications to treatment regimens.

For best results and maximum function restoration, patients are urged to take an active role in their rehabilitation.

CHAPTER EIGHT
RESULTS AND PREDICTION

The purpose of epilepsy surgery is to greatly enhance the quality of life for those with severe, drug-resistant epilepsy.

The type and location of the seizures, the patient's general health, and the success of the surgical procedure are some of the variables that can affect the prognosis and results of epilepsy surgery.

Epilepsy surgery frequently results in a decrease in the frequency and intensity of seizures, and in rare circumstances, it can even be the cause of total seizure independence.

When the source of the epileptic activity is a well-defined, surgically accessible region of the brain, the prognosis is typically better.

A thorough pre-operative assessment, encompassing neuroimaging and electroencephalography (EEG), aids neurosurgeons in precisely identifying the origin of seizures and assessing the viability of surgical intervention.

Long-term studies have demonstrated that a considerable proportion of patients who are good candidates and have successful surgery report a significant improvement in seizure management.

This progress may result in fewer restrictions on day-to-day activities, better cognitive performance, and increased general well-being.

Success Rates As Well As Possible Advantages

The kind of surgery done and the particulars of the patient's epilepsy are two variables that affect the success rates of epilepsy surgery.

When surgery is used to treat focal epilepsies (seizures that originate from a particular location of the brain) as opposed to generalized epilepsies, success rates are often higher.

When surgery is successful and suitable, patients may benefit dramatically in certain circumstances. Seizures may occur less frequently and with less intensity, and there may also be improvements in cognitive function, mood stability, and social relations.

Beyond just controlling seizures, there may be additional advantages such as heightened autonomy and greater participation in everyday activities.

Research has indicated that a notable proportion of people who have surgery for epilepsy see notable enhancements in their quality of life.

Long-term maintenance of this improvement is common, leading to improved psychosocial and general health outcomes.

Hazards And Possible Issues

While there are many advantages to epilepsy surgery, there are also hazards. Patients and their healthcare professionals should carefully examine the potential problems associated with any brain surgery.

Typical dangers include bleeding, infection, and anesthesia-related side effects. There are particular hazards associated with the location of the surgery and the type of brain tissue that will be operated on.

For example, there is a chance that speech, movement, or sensation will be negatively affected by brain surgeries conducted close to important brain regions.

Neurosurgeons assess every patient's condition individually to reduce risks and maximize results. During surgery, sophisticated neuroimaging methods and neurophysiological monitoring assist reduce the risk of problems.

Despite these factors, when epilepsy surgery is carried out by skilled surgical teams in specialized facilities, the overall complication rates are often low.

Enhancements In Life Quality

Enhancing the lives of those with severe, drug-resistant epilepsy is one of the main objectives of epilepsy surgery. Enhancements in life quality have the potential to be significant and diverse.

Many patients find that having surgery to improve seizure control results in fewer limitations on their everyday activities, such as driving or working.

Additionally, it can result in less anxiety related to erratic seizures, better emotional stability, and enhanced cognitive performance.

Patients frequently report improvements in their relationships and social interactions as they become more self-assured in managing their illness.

Enhancements in the individual's quality of life also benefit their family members and caregivers, who frequently feel less stressed and more secure knowing their loved one is more secure from seizures.

Case Studies And Testimonials From Patients

Case studies and patient testimonies offer important insights into how epilepsy surgery affects people and their families in the real world.

These stories frequently describe the process from diagnosis to surgery and beyond, providing insights into the difficulties encountered and the results attained.

Patients report dramatic reductions in seizure frequency or total seizure independence after surgery in numerous published cases.

They frequently describe gains in their capacity to work, interact with people, and pursue interests without having to worry about seizures all the time.

Testimonials from patients also highlight the emotional and psychological changes that can take place when people feel more in charge of their lives.

Case studies are used by healthcare professionals to highlight the range of patient experiences and results, educating other patients and their families about the possible advantages and difficulties of surgery.

Research and Development Continued

Continuous investigation and progress in epilepsy surgery keep expanding the range of available treatments and enhancing patient outcomes.

The main goals of research are to improve pre-operative care, develop new technologies including minimally invasive surgery and responsive neurostimulation, and refine surgical skills.

Ensuring that patients have access to the most cutting-edge treatments available requires clinical trials to assess the efficacy of novel therapies and surgical techniques.

Working together, neurosurgeons, neurologists, and researchers can gain a better knowledge of the fundamental mechanisms driving epilepsy and how best to target them with surgery.

The ultimate goal is to improve seizure control and quality of life outcomes for a variety of populations by making epilepsy surgery more widely available and effective as research advances.

CHAPTER NINE

COMMON QUESTIONS AND ANSWERS

It makes sense that patients and their families would have a lot of questions and worries about epilepsy surgery. When medication fails to manage seizures, one common issue is whether surgery is the best course of action. It's critical to understand that a multidisciplinary team consisting of neurologists, neurosurgeons, and other specialists will usually conduct a thorough review before considering surgery. Finding the precise region of the brain that causes seizures and figuring out whether or not it can be safely removed are the objectives.

The dangers of epilepsy surgery are a further source of worry. There are hazards associated with surgery, like any other procedure: bleeding, infection, and even neurological damage. But these dangers are carefully balanced against the possible advantages of lessening or doing away with seizures. To make an educated choice, patients must thoroughly explore these risks with their healthcare provider.

Patients frequently enquire about the success rates of surgeries for epilepsy. The type of epilepsy, the location of the seizure onset, and the general health of the person can all affect success. In a considerable number of individuals who are suitable candidates, surgery has generally been found to achieve seizure independence or to dramatically reduce the frequency of seizures.

Taking Care Of Often Held Myths And Fears

Medical research has advanced, yet misconceptions and anxieties about surgery for epilepsy linger. The idea that surgery invariably results in serious cognitive or physical deficits is widely held. Although there are hazards associated with surgery, they have been reduced and outcomes have been enhanced by advances in surgical procedures and preoperative examinations. After a successful operation, the majority of patients either feel no change or an improvement in their cognitive performance.

Another concern is that the seizures might get worse after surgery or that the procedure won't properly control the seizures. Reducing seizure frequency and intensity is the main objective of surgery, which is usually considered when medication is not working well to control seizures. The choice to proceed with the surgery is based on careful evaluation and careful consideration of each patient's unique circumstances, however, there are no assurances.

Sometimes, patients are concerned about how their everyday lives will be affected by their recovery. The length of recovery following epilepsy surgery varies based on the kind of procedure and the general health of the patient. Generally speaking, the medical staff will offer comprehensive instructions for postoperative care to facilitate a successful recovery. Patients and their families must keep lines of communication open with their medical team to discuss any worries or unforeseen difficulties that may arise during the healing process.

Faqs Regarding Surgery For Epilepsy

Which kinds of epilepsy are usually candidates for surgical intervention?

When a seizure starts in a particular part of the brain that may be treated or removed, this type of epilepsy is most frequently treated with surgery.

How long does recovery from surgery for epilepsy take?

Recovery periods differ based on the kind of operation and personal circumstances. While some people may heal in a matter of weeks, others could need more time for recuperation and adjustment.

What possible dangers come with having surgery for epilepsy?

Neural impairments, hemorrhage, and infection are among the risks. These hazards are, therefore, carefully balanced against the possible advantages of reducing or eliminating seizures.

Coping Techniques For Families And Patients

Emotional support and practical strategies are also necessary for coping after epilepsy surgery. Family and patients must understand the surgery and its possible consequences. Having a solid support system that includes medical experts, relatives, and friends may be quite helpful while making decisions and during the healing process.

Keeping a journal of seizure activity and any changes in symptoms, following postoperative care recommendations, and being in open communication with healthcare personnel are all important components of developing good coping techniques. Joining support groups or making connections with people who have experienced similar things could also be beneficial for patients. Reassurance and useful guidance can be given by sharing experiences and problem-solving strategies.

A further critical component of adjusting to epilepsy surgery is managing expectations. Although the reduction or elimination of seizures is frequently the aim, individual results may differ. Patients and their families may find it easier to keep a happy attitude and adapt to any changes in seizure control or day-to-day functioning by setting reasonable goals and acknowledging little victories.

Financial And Legal Aspects To Take Into Account

Managing the financial and legal aspects of epilepsy surgery can be challenging, but it's necessary to guarantee complete support and care. It may be necessary for patients and their families to assess health insurance coverage, including the prerequisites for preauthorization of surgical procedures and postoperative care.

Advance directives or powers of attorney are examples of legal considerations that may arise, especially if the procedure carries risks that could impair the patient's ability to make decisions.

If you have any specific questions or concerns, it's best to speak with attorneys who focus on healthcare law.

To control future surgical expenditures, such as hospital stays, surgical fees, rehabilitation, and continuing medical care, financial planning is crucial. Speaking with a healthcare financial counselor or social worker about financial problems can be beneficial for patients as they can offer advice on available options and help programs.

Sources Of Additional Data And Assistance

For patients and families undergoing epilepsy surgery, having access to trustworthy resources and support systems is crucial. Medical professionals who specialize in neurology and neurosurgery can give specific information regarding surgical alternatives, risks, and anticipated results depending on the patient's situation.

For patients and their families, national and local epilepsy foundations frequently provide educational materials, support groups, and internet tools. These groups can be a great resource for learning about epilepsy surgery, making connections with people who are going through similar things, and getting access to legal and advocacy resources.

Furthermore, social media sites and online forums could offer chances to get in touch with others who have had epilepsy surgery or are thinking about getting one. Throughout the process, exchanging experiences and insights can provide comfort, useful guidance, and emotional support.

www.ingramcontent.com/pod-product-compliance
Lightning Source LLC
Chambersburg PA
CBHW071842210526
45479CB00001B/259